This bite-sized book has been designed to give you a useful overview of winter wellbeing and to help you achieve the following:

- Take personal responsibility for your wellbeing
- Keep active and embrace the change of season
- Sustain a balanced and healthy lifestyle
- Look after your mental health and feel happier
- Be kind and care for other people

Please note that this bite-sized book is in no way meant to replace the advice of a medical professional, however it does offer some useful suggestions that may well help you.

GW00645159

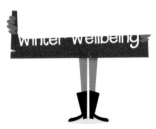

3

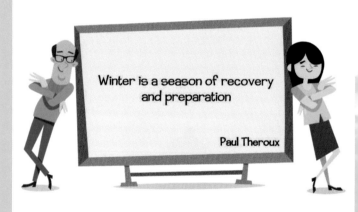

Winter is a season of recovery and preparation

Paul Theroux

Winter wellbeing

Winter can sometimes be a challenging time for people both mentally and physically. You may find yourself becoming more susceptible to all sorts of bugs and blues. It can also be the time of year when you fall into the trap of eating comfort foods and overindulging.

It can be tempting to want to stay inside and hibernate, however it is important to get lots of fresh air and exercise even when it is cold outside. Being proactive and responsible for your health and well-being will help you to feel better through the winter season.

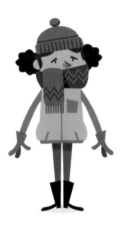

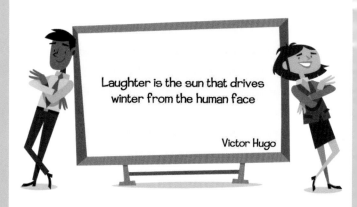

Laughter is the sun that drives winter from the human face

Victor Hugo

What happens when it's cold?

Cold weather can be harmful, especially for older people. It can weaken the immune system, increase blood pressure, thicken the blood and lower body temperature. This can increase the risk of high blood pressure, heart attacks, strokes, and chest infections.

It is therefore important to take special care of yourself and keep warm.

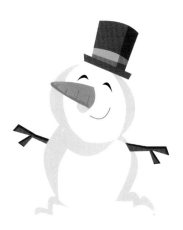

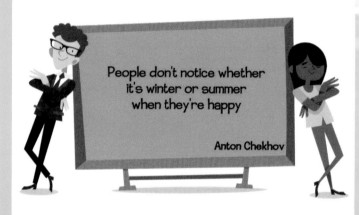

People don't notice whether
it's winter or summer
when they're happy

Anton Chekhov

Being at your best

Winter is a time when you can let your wellbeing habits slide, if you are not careful. Faced with shorter days, less natural light and colder temperatures, it can be easy to slip into unhelpful lifestyle patterns and neglect your wellbeing.

This is the time when you need to put some extra effort into your self-care and cultivate healthy habits so you can feel well.

Here are some useful tips to help you to be at your best this winter:

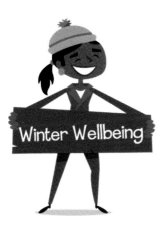

How to
be well in
the winter

Winter and sunshine

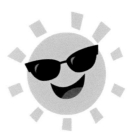

Your circadian rhythm is your 24-hour internal clock that is running in the background of your brain and cycles between sleepiness and alertness at regular intervals. It's also known as your sleep/wake cycle.

We all need sunshine to help our mind and body to wake up and trigger normal bodily function.

A lack of sunlight can make you feel sluggish and tired. Getting enough sunlight can be challenging during the winter months, particularly if you work long hours inside during the day.

Any opportunity you can take to get outside and put your face up to the sky will give you a healthy boost. Getting outside as much as you can during the daytime in the winter and exposing yourself to natural daylight can be very helpful. Even when the sun isn't shining!

Seasonal Affective Disorder

Seasonal Affective Disorder (SAD) is sometimes known as "winter depression" because the symptoms are usually more apparent and more severe during this time of year.

Some of the symptoms of SAD can include:

- A persistent low mood
- A loss of pleasure or interest in normal everyday activities
- Irritability
- Feelings of despair, guilt and worthlessness
- Feeling lethargic and sleepy during the day
- Finding it extra hard to get up in the morning
- Craving carbohydrates and gaining weight

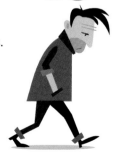

For some people, these symptoms can be severe and have a significant impact on their day-to-day activities.

Let the light shine in!

Because you may be exposed to less light and sunshine during the winter months, light therapy can be effective for seasonal depression.

A good way to get light therapy at home in the winter is to sit in front of a light box for 30–60 minutes each day.

Light boxes give out very bright light at least 10 times stronger than ordinary home and workplace lighting.

Something else that may be helpful is a dawn simulator as a bedside light. This can be connected to your alarm clock and mimics sunrise and wakes you up gradually.

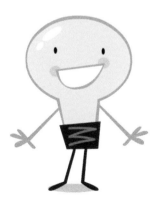

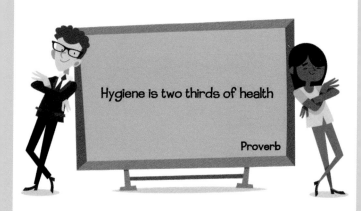

Hygiene is two thirds of health

Proverb

Wash your hands

With more bugs about at this time of year, it is extremely important to wash your hands often and well. You need to do this especially before eating as this is one of the easiest ways to help prevent the spread of infections.

Follow these four steps every time you wash your hands.

- Wet your hands with clean, running water, and apply soap
- Lather your hands with the soap for at least 20 seconds
- Clean the backs of your hands and between your fingers
- Rinse and dry your hands thoroughly

NB – In the winter especially it is also a good idea to carry antibacterial hand wipes or a small bottle of sanitiser.

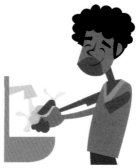

15

Get rid of used tissues

If you have a cold and you use paper tissues throw them away after each use rather than keep using the same one. The germs will continue to transfer to your hands.

Remember that most flu viruses and cold germs can live up to twelve hours on a tissue!

Also make sure that you don't leave them lying around to avoid spreading your germs to other people.

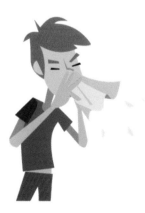

Get a flu jab

Flu can be really unpleasant, however if you are otherwise fit and healthy it will usually clear up on its own within a week or so.

Flu can be more severe in certain people including:

- Anyone aged 65 and over
- Pregnant women
- Children and adults with an underlying health condition (such as long-term heart or respiratory disease)
- Children and adults with weakened immune systems

It is highly recommended that you have a flu vaccine every year and for those in these risk categories flu vaccinations are available on the NHS.

This is to help protect adults and children at risk of flu and its complications. If you are not eligible you can speak to your pharmacist about how you can pay for one of these and where to receive the treatment.

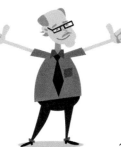

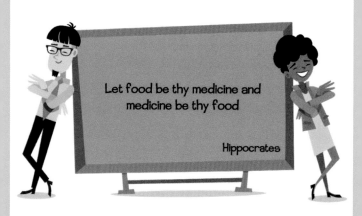

Let food be thy medicine and medicine be thy food

Hippocrates

Eat yourself healthy

You can really protect your immune system by eating healthy food. Certain foods like garlic, lemon, ginger, tomatoes and onions are all great for warding off colds. Plenty of fruit and fresh vegetables will provide you with antioxidants and a whole host of vitamins and minerals.

So let healthy food be your medicine!

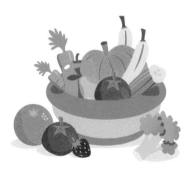

Reduce sugar

Eating or drinking 100 grams (8 teaspoons) of refined sugar, the equivalent of one 12-ounce can of sugary fizzy drink soda, can reduce the ability of white blood cells to kill germs by 40%. The immune-suppressing effect of refined sugar starts less than thirty minutes after ingestion and may last for five hours.

When it's cold it can be very tempting to reach out for those comfort foods and get a quick sugar fix. Before you do however, stop and remind yourself what it is doing to your immune system. This is the time of year it really needs all the help it can get.

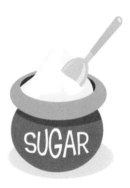

Boost your vitamins

Vitamin C is at the top of the list among natural immune boosters for your body. The research on the immune boosting properties of the vitamin has been extensive and eating lots of delicious seasonal fruit and vegetables will help.

Vitamin D is also known as the sunshine vitamin, and is produced by the body as a response to sun exposure; it can also be consumed in food or supplements. Having enough vitamin D is important for maintaining healthy bones and teeth.

Most people can make enough vitamin D from sun exposure during the summer, however synthesis can be inadequate in the winter.

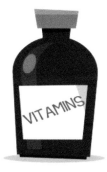

Explore supplements

Taking the herbal remedy Echinacea, according to some research, can more than halve the risk of catching a common cold. It is made from nine species of herbaceous plants in the family Asteraceae which are commonly called purple coneflower. It is available as liquid, tablets and delicious herbal teas.

It is well worth visiting your pharmacist or health store to discuss which supplements may work best for you.

Also discuss with your doctor first if you are taking any medication as some supplements can interfere with these.

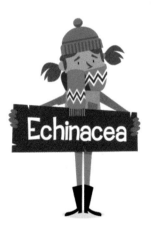

Get walking

To keep your immune system healthy, exercise is one of the best things that you can do. Wrap up warm and go for a lovely big walk. This is even better than going to the gym because you will get lots of fresh air and natural daylight. The cooler weather is great to invigorate and stimulate the senses.

You may want to measure and track your steps for added motivation and aim to walk 10,000 steps a day.

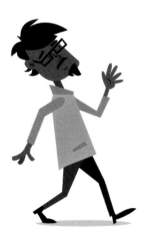

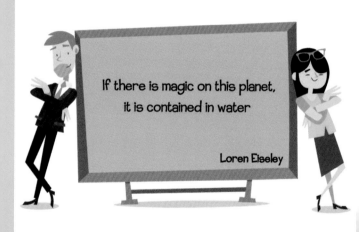

If there is magic on this planet,
it is contained in water

Loren Eiseley

Keep hydrated

Water may not be the drink of choice in the winter, however keeping hydrated is one of the best things that you can do to keep healthy and it is vital for all bodily functions. An important part of flushing out bacteria is the actual flushing!

Be planet friendly and use a reusable bottle and keep it with you at all times. Keep reminders around to ensure that you are drinking water throughout the day.

By keeping hydrated you will feel more alert and energised. There are also lots of delicious herbal teas available and these will also add to your recommended quota of around two litres a day.

There are over a billion people on this planet who don't have access to clean drinking water. We are extremely fortunate that we do!

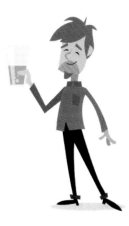

Manage stress

Stress is often cited as a nasty precursor to deflating your immune system and leaving you more vulnerable to viruses. If you are feeling rundown and overstretched it is time to slow down, sharpen your stress management skills and strengthen your immunity.

For more tips on avoiding burnout and managing stress please access the free online Life Skills Library detailed at the back of this book.

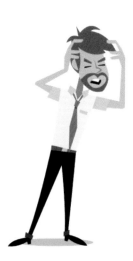

Sleep well

When we get less sunlight our serotonin levels automatically fall. This can lead to you having less energy and fewer positive feelings. As a result you can naturally be more tired and low during the winter.

A good night's rest is one of the best ways to boost your immune system and also to make you feel better and more energised. The quality of your sleep is very important and preparation for bedtime can be really helpful.

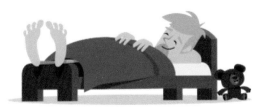

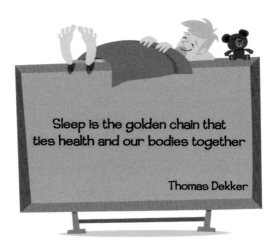

Sleep is the golden chain that
ties health and our bodies together

Thomas Dekker

Create a sanctuary for sleep

Here are some useful tips to create a sanctuary for sleep:

- Declutter your bedroom and keep it tidy
- Get a pillow spray such as lavender and geranium to help with sleep
- Make sure that your bedroom is the right temperature, somewhere between 16°C and 18°C (60°F to 65°F)
- Avoid mobile technology in the bedroom and get a separate alarm clock
- Block out any light as this is essential for sleep and the absence of light sends a critical signal to your body that it is time to rest
- Focus on breathing deeply and count your blessings and the things you are grateful for, one by one, as you drift off to sleep

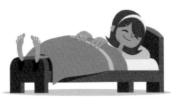

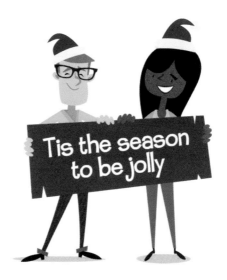

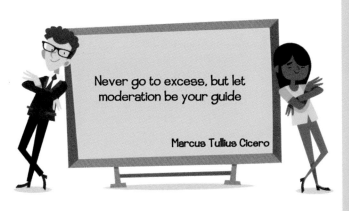

Never go to excess, but let moderation be your guide

Marcus Tullius Cicero

Be alcohol aware

Despite the fact that it is the season to be jolly, excessive alcohol consumption can cause harm to your body's immune system in two ways.

First of all it can produce an overall nutritional deficiency, depriving your body of valuable immune boosting nutrients.

Secondly, alcohol, like sugar, consumed in excess can reduce the ability of white blood cells to kill germs and deplete your body of vitamin B, which can make you depressed.

Alcohol, despite the association with celebrations, is best enjoyed in moderation with the maximum recommended guidelines being 14 units a week for both men and women.

It is also recommended to have a minimum of 2 alcohol-free days a week.

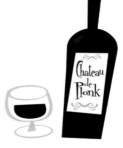

Manage your social media

FOMO has been recognised as an emerging psychological disorder brought on by the advance of technology. It is an acronym standing for the expression fear of missing out. This is used to describe that feeling of anxiety which many people experience when they discover that other people are having fun together or are being successful at something.

If you do decide to use social media over the festive season, avoid comparing your experience to those of your friends. Remember that most people only share the best bits of their lives online and you don't know what is going on behind the smiling selfies.

Life is a lot easier when you don't concern yourself with what everybody else is doing.

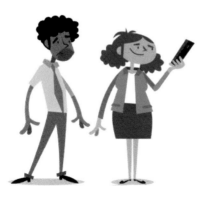

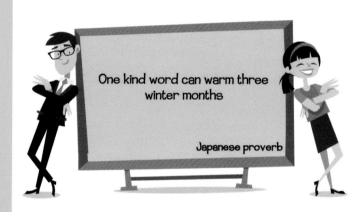

One kind word can warm three winter months

Japanese proverb

Support others

The festive season, for many, can be a time of celebration, fun and togetherness. It is also important to remember that Christmas can also be a challenging time for some.

For those who spend Christmas alone it can be difficult and isolating. It is so important to think of ways to help other people by being kind and thoughtful.

This is a time you could consider volunteering. Various research has shown that giving something back can help you feel good about yourself too. So you may want to consider how you can help other people.

Looking out for elderly people who may need support or offering company to people who are lonely is the best gift you can give.

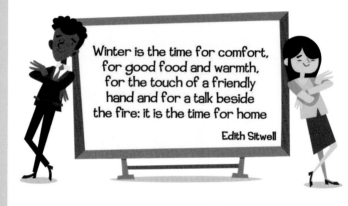

Winter is the time for comfort, for good food and warmth, for the touch of a friendly hand and for a talk beside the fire: it is the time for home

Edith Sitwell

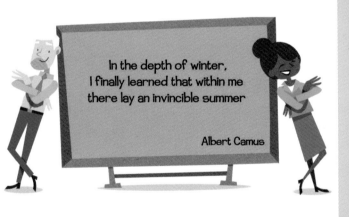

In the depth of winter,
I finally learned that within me
there lay an invincible summer

Albert Camus

If you are looking for more in-depth advice these websites are very helpful and have been curated for the excellent advice they offer around winter wellbeing:

1. www.nhs.uk/live-well/healthy-body/five-ways-to-stay-healthy-this-winter

2. www.ageuk.org.uk/information-advice/health-wellbeing/keep-well-this-winter

3. www.simplyhealth.co.uk/sh/pages/healthy-you/winter-wellness

4. www.cclg.org.uk/WinterWellbeing

5. www.mentalhealth.org.uk/blog/tis-season-be-jolly

6. www.nhs.uk/live-well/healthy-body/keep-warm-keep-well

7. www.nhs.uk/live-well/healthy-body/10-winter-illnesses

8. www.nhs.uk/staywell

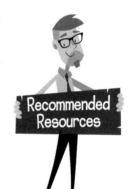

Recommended Resources